PLACEMENT OF EKG LEADS:

I0482690

Right and left arm leads should be placed outwardly on the shoulders (preferentially over bone rather than muscle)

V4 should be placed in the fifth intercostal space on the mid-clavicular line

V1 and V2 are positioned in the fourth intercostal space

V3 lies halfway between V2 and V4

V4, V5 and V6 should be placed along a horizontal line — this line does not necessarily follow the intercostal space

RA   LA

V1   V2
      V3
     V4 V5 V6

Anterior axilla line

Mid-axilla line

C

RL   LL

The right leg lead (ground lead) should be placed below the umbilicus

The left leg lead should be just below the umbilicus

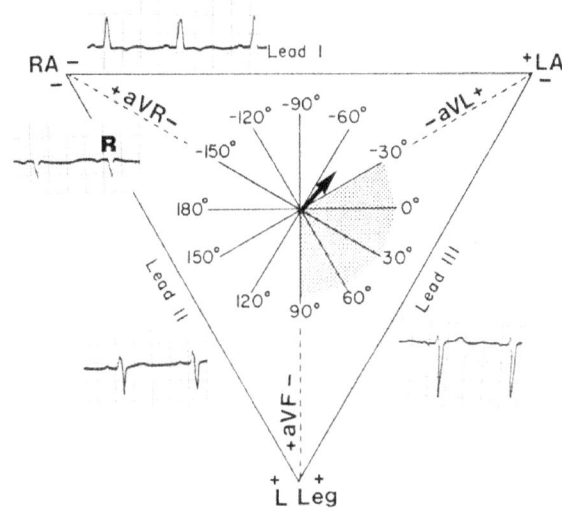

Learning to interpret 12 Lead EKG's does not have to be a daunting task. Some find the learning a painful and "head aching" venture. However once you understand the basic rules it is little more than repetition. In this book there are nearly 100 real 12 Lead EKG's. Take your time with each and you will be flying through 12 Leads in no time.

First:

A. Label the 12 Lead at how it identifies the section of the heart.

1. Lead I: High Lateral
2. Lead II: Inferior
3. Lead III: Inferior
4. AVR: Lead II mirror.
5. AVL: High Lateral
6. AVF: Inferior
7. V1: Septal

8. V2: Septal
9. V3: Anterior
10. V4: Anterior
11. V5: Low Lateral
12. V6: Low Lateral

We have a memory aid to learn how to label the 12 Lead:

All Asses **I**n **I**raq **I**ncluding **L**ittle **H**abib are a **L**ittle **H**arry

When you start labeling the 12 Lead EKG go from right to left spelling out your memory

aid. Oh…don't get offended by the memory aid, I came up with that while in Iraq with

my Iraq counterparts who called me Habib…*they thought it was hilarious.*

Second:

B. Circle all signs of ectopy, elevation, ischemia, , or irregularities.

1. You don't have to circle everything if there is a lot but give yourself plenty

examples.

Medicsmi

C. Write down the areas that you have circled from identified issues in the EKG.

   1. "Q" waves must be at least 2/3 the size of the "RS" complexes to be considered an active MI.

   2. Damage or ischemia must be shown in at least 2 contiguous leads to be an active MI.

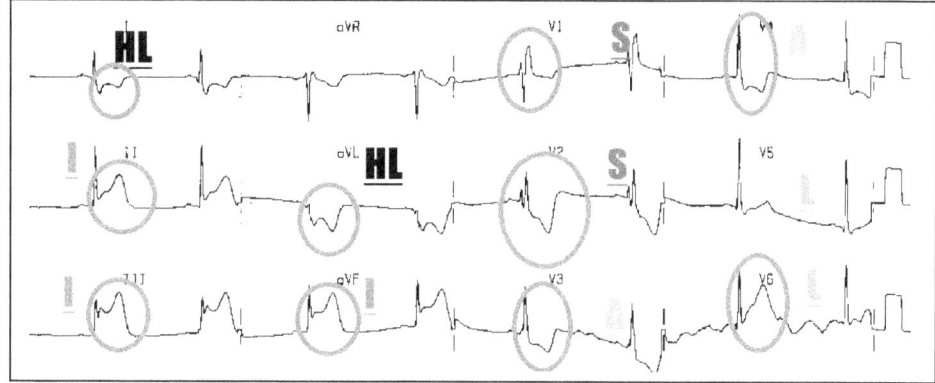

a. Inferior ST elevation

b. High Lateral Ischemia

c. Septal Ischemia

d. Anterior Ischemia

e. Diagnosis: Inferior & Lateral Wall AMI

blank

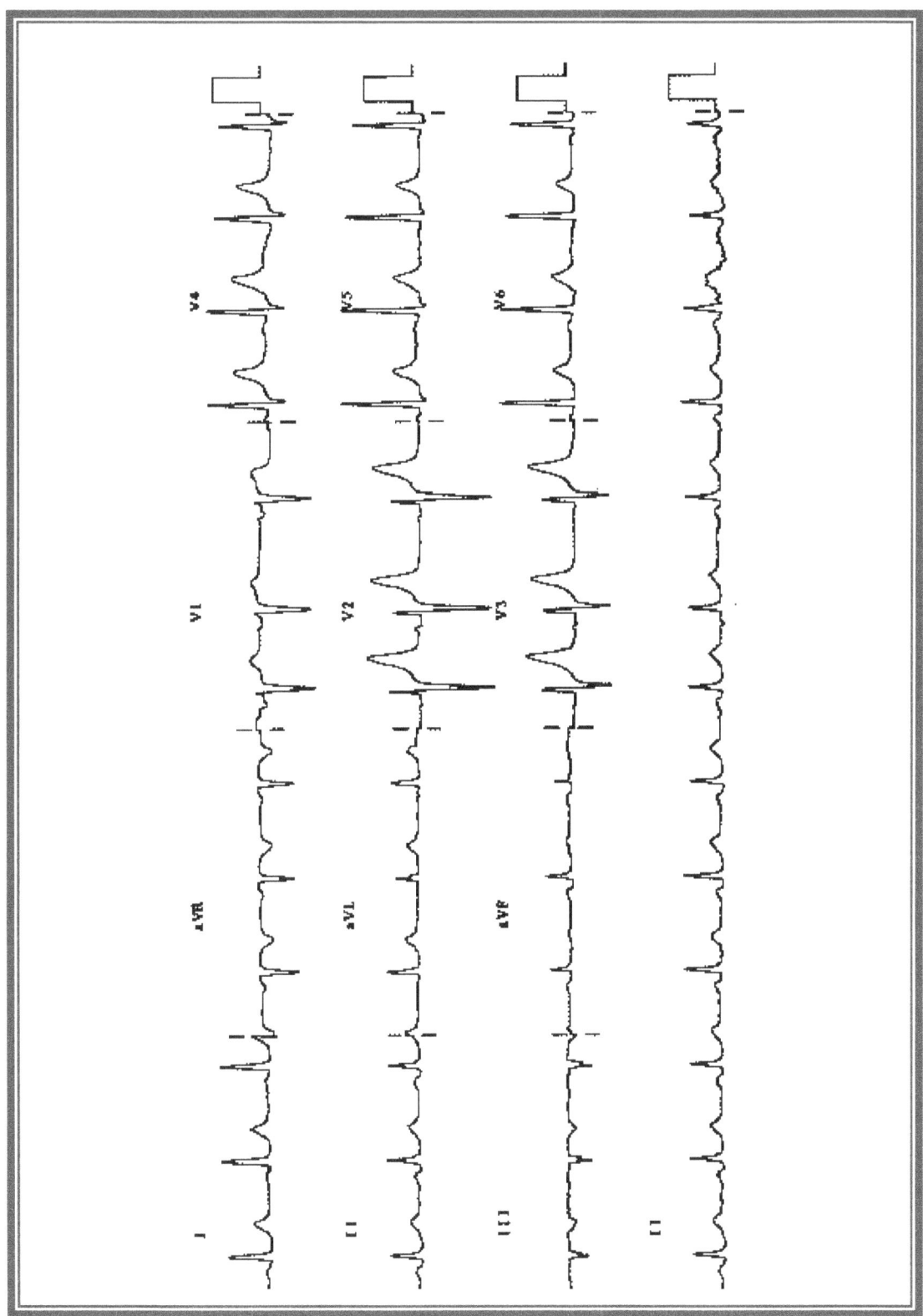

Write the Diagnosis of the previous EKG's:

1._____

2._____

3._____

blank

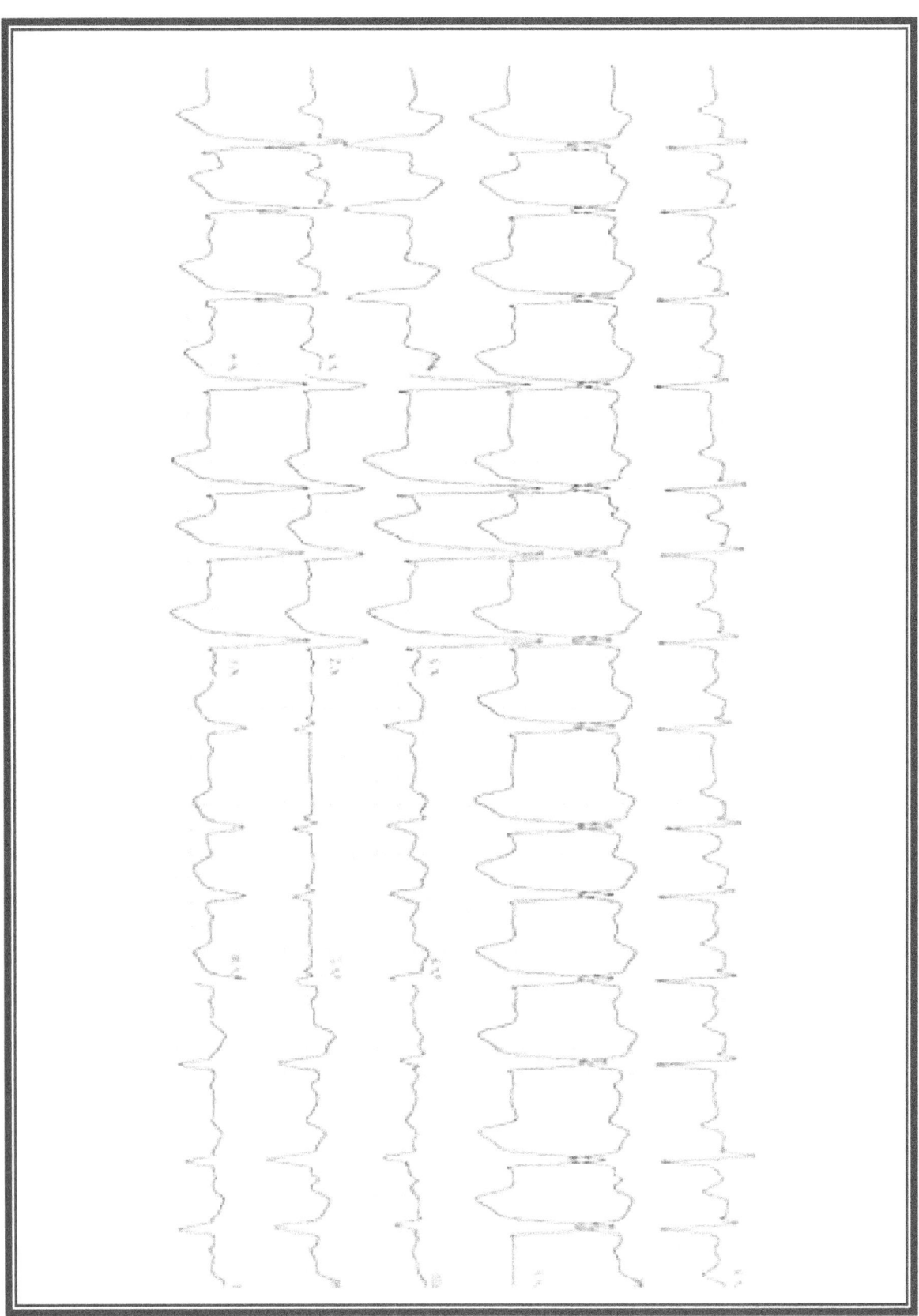

Write the Diagnosis of the previous EKG's:

1._____

2._____

3._____

4._____

5._____

6._____

7._____

8._____

9._____

10._____

11._____

12._____

13._____

14._____

15._____

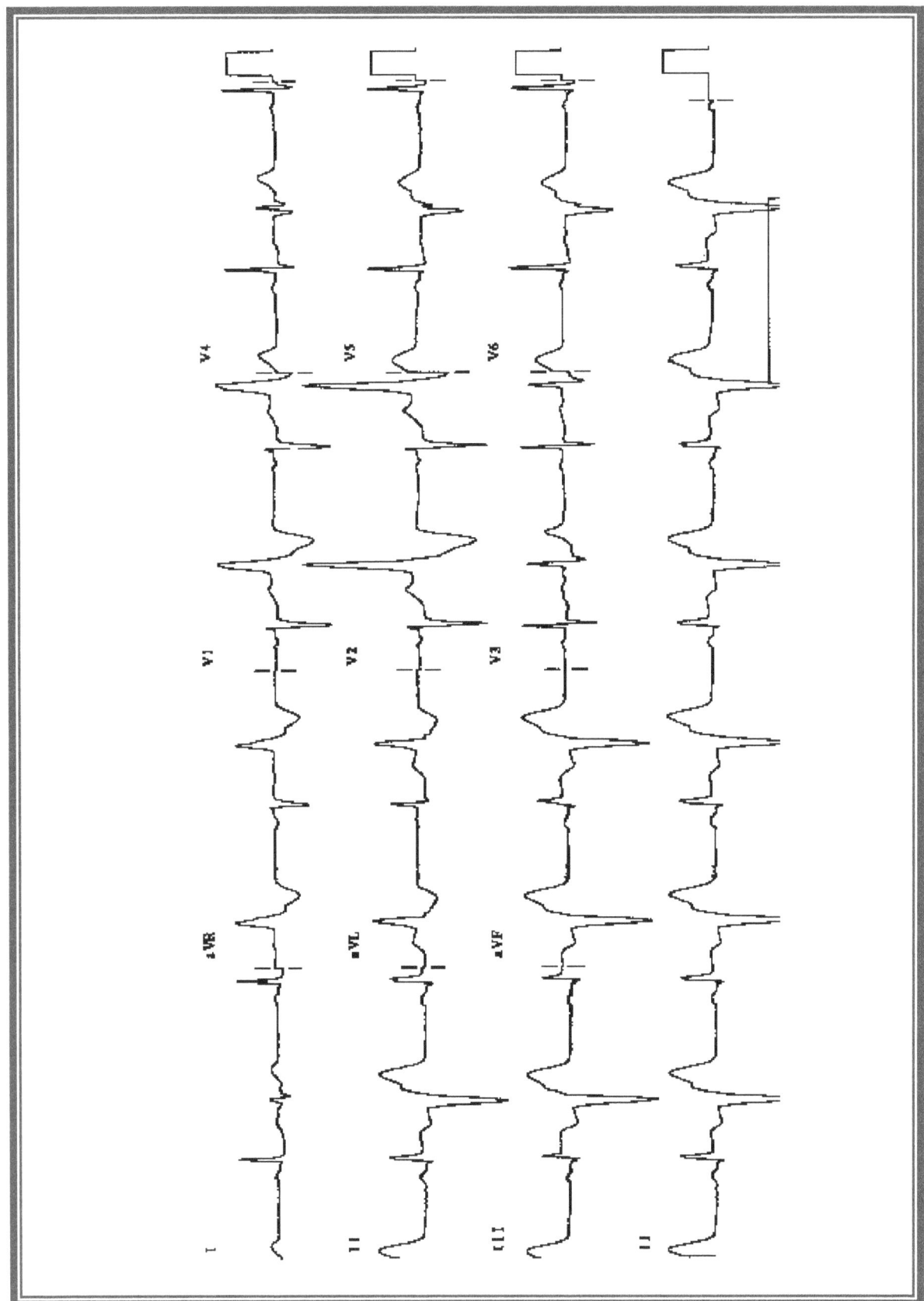

Write the Diagnosis of the previous EKG's:

1._____

2._____

3._____

4._____

5._____

6._____

7._____

8._____

9._____

10._____

11._____

12._____

13._____

14._____

15._____

16._____

17._____

blank

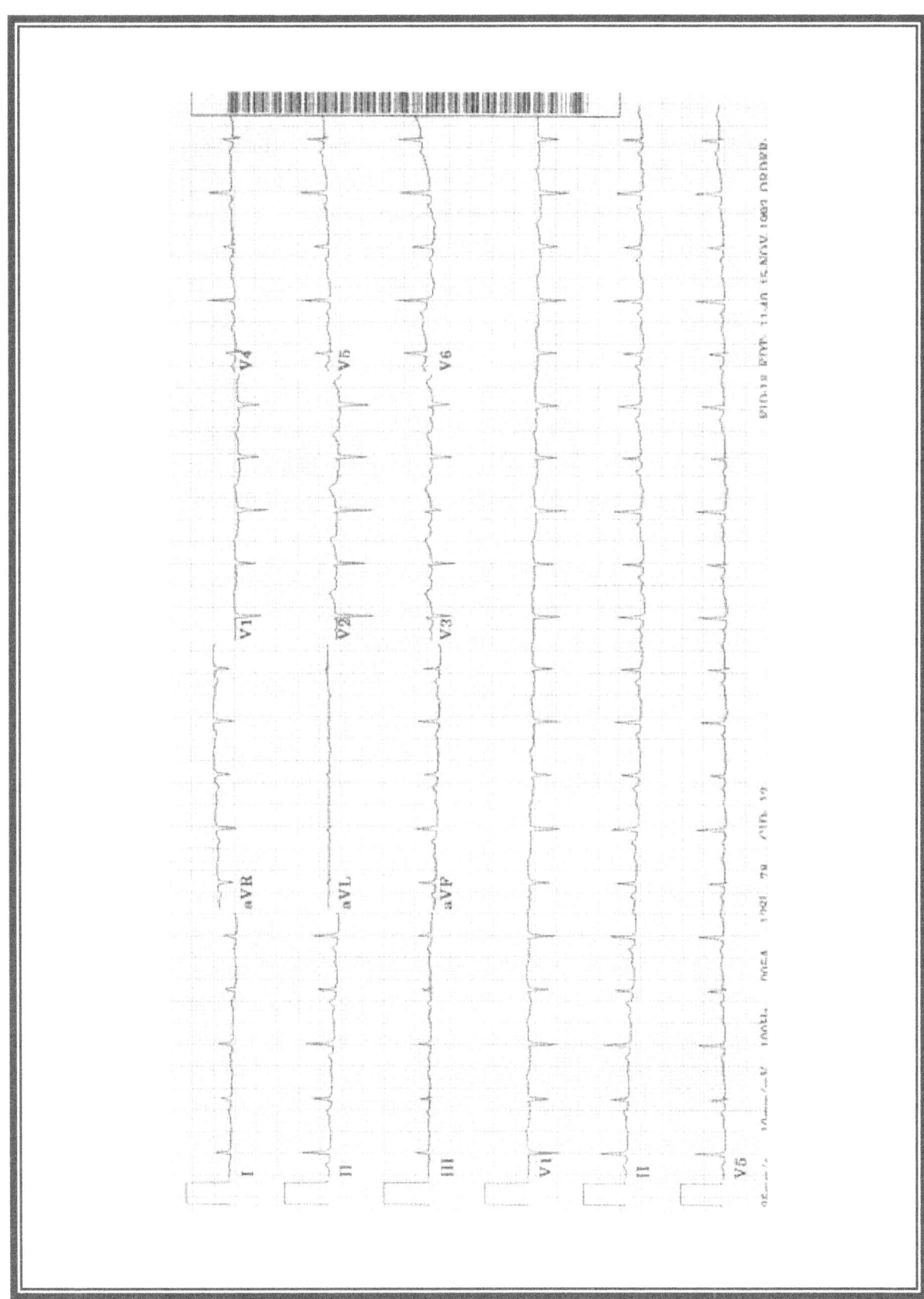

Write the Diagnosis of the previous EKG's:

1._____

2._____

3._____

4._____

5._____

6._____

7._____

8._____

9._____

10._____

11._____

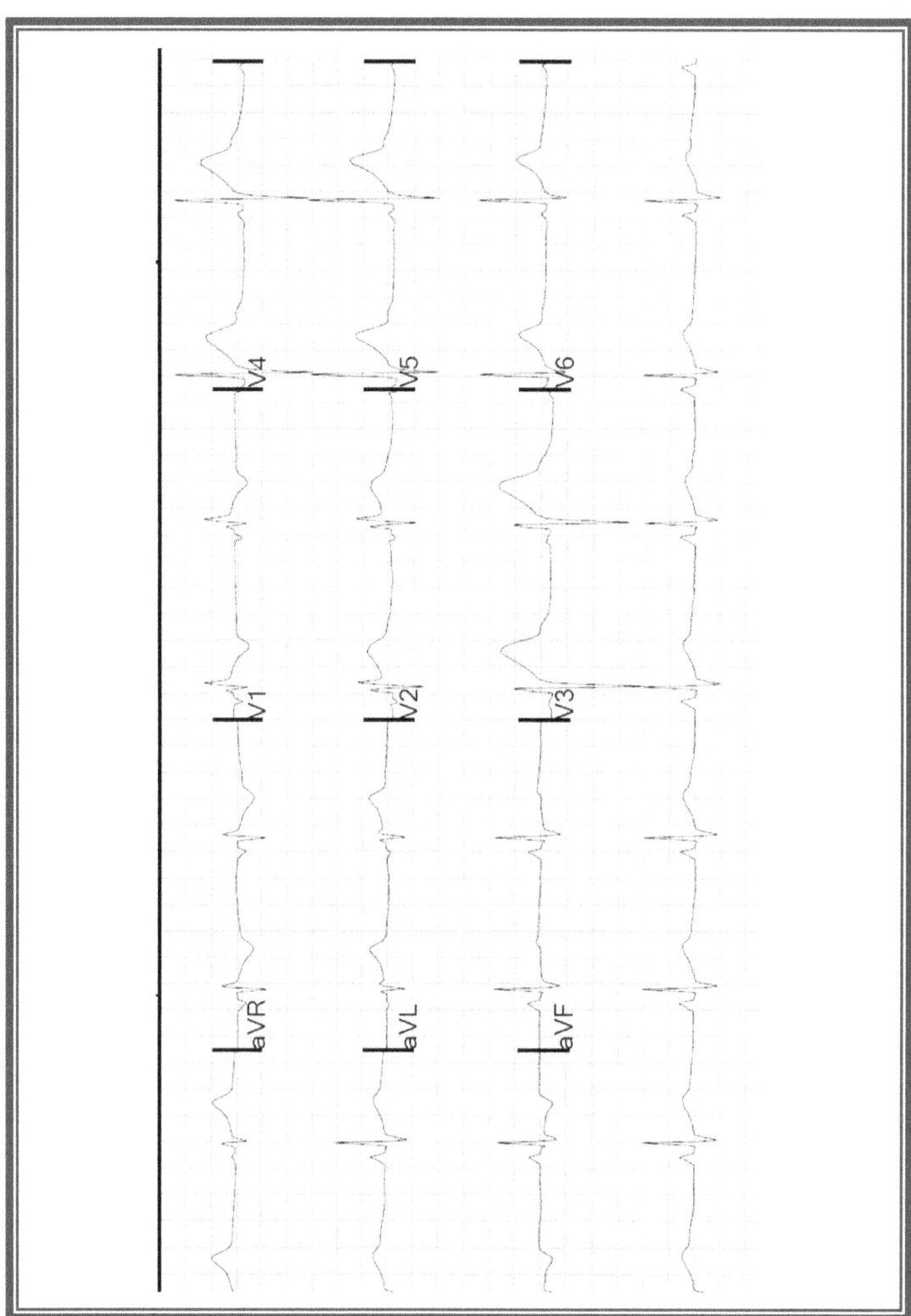

Write the Diagnosis of the previous EKG's:

1._____

2._____

3._____

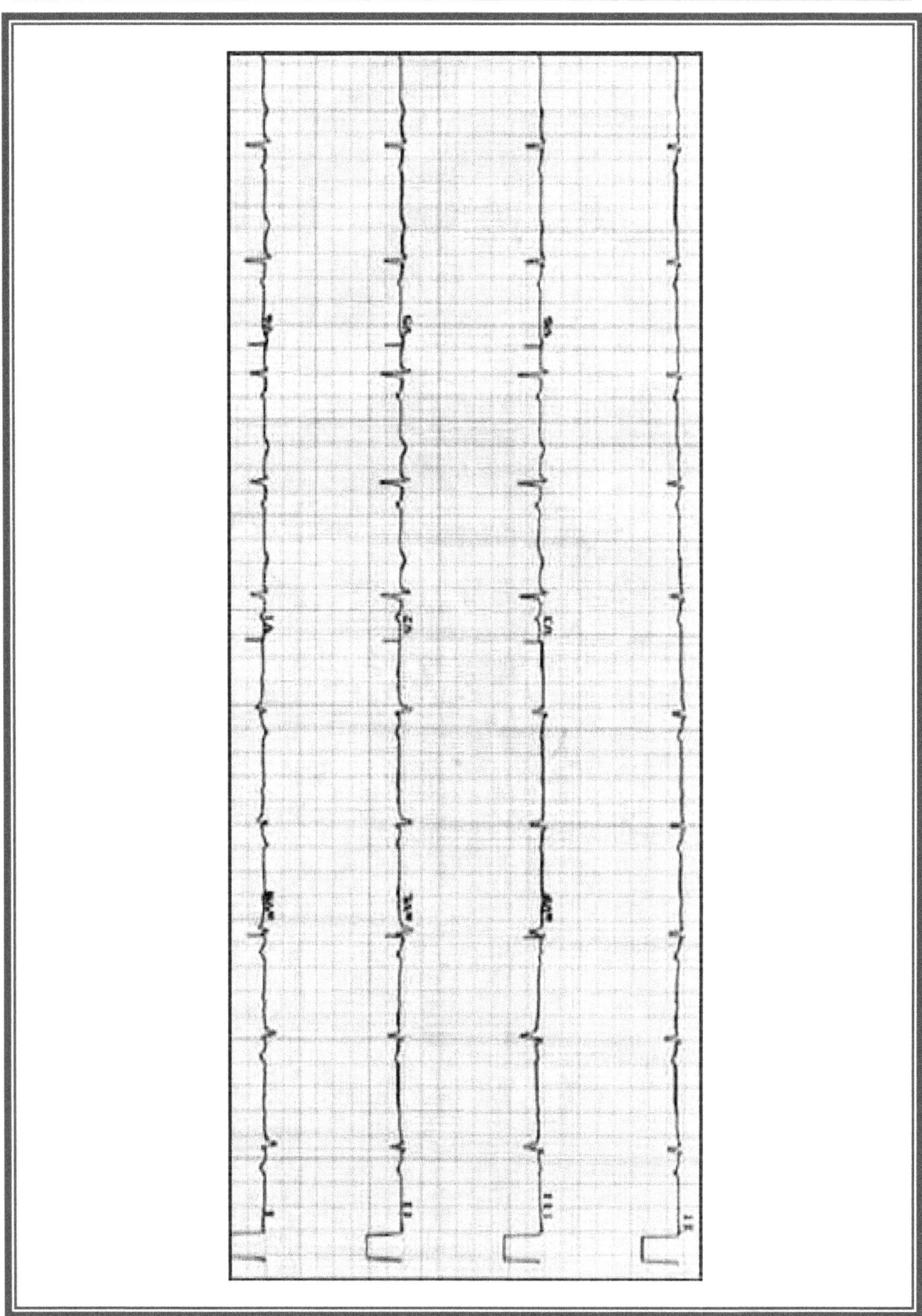

WRITE THE DIAGNOSIS OF THE PREVIOUS EKG'S:

1. _____

2. _____

3. _____

4. _____

5. _____

6. _____

7. _____

8. _____

9. _____

10. _____

11. _____

12. _____

13. _____

14. _____

15. _____

16. _____

17. _____

18. _____

19. _____

20. _____

21. _____

22. _____

23. _____

24. _____

25. _____

WRITE THE DIAGNOSIS OF THE PREVIOUS EKG'S:

26. _____

27. _____

28. _____

29. _____

30. _____

31. _____

32. _____

33. _____

34. _____

35. _____

36. _____

37. _____

38. _____

CHECK OUT:

12 LEAD EKG IN ABOUT AN HOUR!

*AVAILABLE BOTH PAPERBACK AND ELECTRONIC.

www.ingramcontent.com/pod-product-compliance
Lightning Source LLC
Chambersburg PA
CBHW080307180526
45167CB00006B/2709